Beyond Straight Teeth:
A Consumer's Guide
to Orthodontics

On the cover: One of our many satisfied patients, Laura Roberson, an accomplished equestrian who was treated with the *Bio-Esthetic Smile Design System* found exclusively at White Orthodontics.

Beyond Straight Teeth: A Consumer's Guide to Orthodontics

Paul R White DDS

ISBN: 151865360X
ISBN 13: 9781518653605

Table of Contents

Introduction · vii

Why Are Straight Teeth So Important? · · · · · · · · · · · · · · 1

Finding an Orthodontist: The *Right* Choice Makes
all the Difference · 22

Beyond Straight Teeth · 35

A Matter of Life and Breath · · · · · · · · · · · · · · · · · · · 57

Paying for Orthodontics · 75

What's New in Orthodontics? · · · · · · · · · · · · · · · · · · 83

Let the Journey Begin! · 95

Fun Facts about Smiles · 97

Introduction

Have you ever noticed what the attractive television anchor, the handsome actor, the perky cheerleader, or the alluring model all have in common? They all have a beautiful smile. Studies have shown that people with an attractive smile are more successful personally as well as professionally than those with crooked teeth or an unattractive smile. The bottom line is that when you feel good about yourself, you have more confidence. Samuel Johnson once said, "Self-confidence is the first requisite to great undertakings."

Unfortunately, most of us are not born with a beautiful smile, and that's where orthodontics can be essential.

When choosing an orthodontist, it's important to understand that not all orthodontic experiences or outcomes are the same. Just as two chefs can start with the same "ingredients" and one can create an exquisite, gourmet meal while the other can make the toughest piece of "shoe leather" you've ever tried to eat, two orthodontists can end up with quite different results even though they may use the same appliances. There are numerous factors that contribute to these discrepancies, ranging from the training, philosophy, and ability of the orthodontist to the talent, training, and passion of the orthodontic team and finally the technology and materials employed during orthodontic treatment. Most people seeking orthodontic treatment rely on their general dentist for guidance. However, most dentists have had little to no orthodontic training, and their opinions may not be valid. A recent survey of the orthodontic referral patterns of general dentists revealed that the most important criteria in determining to which orthodontist they refer their patients is location—hardly a ringing endorsement of the orthodontist. While I realize that orthodontics is not a life-or-death situation, can you imagine if your son or daughter had a brain tumor and your pediatrician recommended the closest neurosurgeon?

After consulting with over ten thousand patients regarding their orthodontic care, I've come to the conclusion that patients are confused and that many times it's the orthodontists who are causing the confusion. Unfortunately, unlike the medical profession, there is a lack of consensus among the orthodontic profession as to a specific protocol for a particular diagnosis. In fact, there are times we can't even agree on a diagnosis! The goal of this book is to help you navigate through the confusion, misinformation, and bias regarding orthodontics that you may encounter at the dentist, surfing the web, on the soccer field, or even among different orthodontists. Orthodontic treatment can have a profoundly positive effect on your self-esteem and your health, but it must be done properly, so I applaud your decision to find out more! After completing this book, you'll have all the information you need to make a sound decision regarding orthodontics for you or for someone in your family. Enjoy!

Why Are Straight Teeth So Important?

Your smile is the first thing that other people notice about you. It reflects how you feel about yourself to those around you. When you have crowded or misaligned teeth, your whole appearance is affected and your positive attributes can be overshadowed by an unattractive smile. You've heard it said that you never get a second chance to make a first impression. In fact, groundbreaking research from Princeton psychologists Janine Willis and Alexander Todorov revealed that all it takes is a tenth of a second to form an impression of a stranger from their face. Like it or not, judgments based on facial appearance play a powerful role in how we treat others and how we get treated. Psychologists have long known that attractive people get better outcomes in practically all walks of life. Whether it is a child facing the rigors of adolescence or an adult concerned about their appearance, an attractive smile always creates a better impression from the outside as well as from the inside.

In addition to the obvious social concerns associated with an unattractive smile, there are also significant health challenges with crooked teeth and an improper bite. Crowded teeth are obviously more difficult to clean, which can lead to periodontal, or gum, disease. According to the American Academy of Periodontology, people with periodontal disease are almost twice as likely to have heart disease.

A malocclusion is literally a bad bite. The incidence of malocclusion has been estimated to be 55–60 percent of the population. An improper bite places undue stress on the teeth and the supporting structures, creating tooth shifting, premature tooth wear, and gum recession. Furthermore, abfractions can develop. An abfraction is a loss of tooth structure that is not caused by tooth decay, located along the gum line. In extreme cases, tooth loss can occur. Gum disease, which usually results from poor oral hygiene, is still a leading cause of tooth loss among adults. However, I meet with adults every day who have excellent oral hygiene but who are still in danger of losing their teeth due to excessive tooth wear and bone loss from an improper bite. You can just imagine their frustration! It can take years and years and cost tens of thousands of dollars for a dentist to restore a damaged mouth back to health with crowns or caps, whereas a well-treated orthodontic case can give a patient a healthy and *natural* smile for life!

Another consequence of an unhealthy bite is temporomandibular dysfunction, otherwise known as TMD or TMJ. When the teeth are not properly aligned and coordinated with a stable jaw position, the jaw can be dislocated when chewing. The jaw muscles are constantly contracted to maintain this unstable jaw position, which places stress on the jaw muscles and within the jaw joint itself, leading to

TMJ. As a result, problems can develop with the muscles (myofascial pain) or in the joint (internal derangement). Some signs of an internal derangement are clicking or popping, jaw locking, grating noises in front of the ear where the joint is located, tinnitus, or ringing in the ears and vertigo or dizziness. Patients with overworked jaw muscles can experience fatigue when chewing, limited opening of the mouth, and most commonly headaches and neck aches. The incidence of TMD in the general population is approximately 6–12 percent and is most commonly seen in women between the ages of twenty-five and thirty-five. However, I have treated patients as young as eleven years of age for TMD; therefore, every patient should be screened for TMJ dysfunction prior to beginning any orthodontic treatment.

It's also important to note that orthodontics, if not done properly, can contribute to TMJ problems. Interestingly, the majority of the patients that I treat for TMJ have worn braces at least once, yet we use a specific type of orthodontic treatment known as *functional* orthodontics to relieve their pain and headaches.

Do I Need Braces?

For some people the need for orthodontic treatment is obvious; for others the need for braces is more subtle. Basically, people choose to have orthodontics to improve aesthetics, function, or both. Most people seeking orthodontic treatment are usually concerned with the alignment of their teeth and are seeking to improve their smile by straightening their teeth, and that is a great reason for wearing braces. However, you may be surprised to learn that there is a much more important reason to have orthodontics—correcting your bite. As I mentioned previously, a malocclusion, or improper bite, can lead to premature tooth wear, gum recession, crowding of the teeth, headaches, neck aches, and TMD (temporomandibular dysfunction). Several years ago, *Compendium*, a dental journal, stated that the most *under*diagnosed disease of the oral cavity is occlusal attrition (premature tooth wear).

What's the *Right Time*?

 It's never too late to change your smile. The biology for moving teeth is the same for adults as it is for children and teenagers. You've probably

noticed more adults undergoing orthodontic treatment either to improve their smile or to correct their bite. Today's health-conscious adults have found aesthetic treatment options, such as clear braces, hidden braces placed on the inside of the teeth, and a "brace-less" option known as Invisalign, to achieve a beautiful smile without the embarrassment of wearing metal braces.

In growing children, the need for orthodontic treatment may not be apparent to the untrained eye. It's not uncommon for a young child to have well-aligned front teeth yet not have sufficient room for the remaining permanent teeth to erupt. In the upper jaw, the canines, or "eye" teeth, are the most commonly blocked permanent teeth during development. In certain instances, these teeth may become impacted or stuck and require surgical exposure followed by orthodontic traction to bring them into their proper position. As a matter of fact, about 30 percent of developing upper canines may become impacted. Fortunately, if detected early, interceptive orthodontic treatment can create sufficient space for the erupting canines and significantly reduce the incidence of impaction. As part of their education, orthodontic specialists are trained in the growth and development of the jaws and can detect problems with tooth eruption or jaw growth.

Early Treatment (Interceptive Orthodontics)

Like most diseases, early detection and treatment of a malocclusion is usually the most effective approach. And as with many diseases, if left untreated, a malocclusion usually becomes worse with time. While a malocclusion can be corrected at any age, an early evaluation and treatment can help patients avoid the problems associated with a malocclusion. Early treatment, or interceptive orthodontics, has gained popularity over the last ten to fifteen years as our understanding of facial growth and development has improved. Unlike in years past when orthodontic treatment was delayed until all of the permanent teeth were erupted, early treatment is usually initiated before all the baby teeth are lost. The most ideal time to start interceptive orthodontics is after the permanent front teeth have erupted and before the primary (baby) molars become loose. So what's the right age? The American Association of Orthodontists recommends that every child have an orthodontic evaluation by age seven. In some instances, especially with boys, that may be a bit too soon. But I would suggest that once the upper front teeth are erupted, it's time to see an orthodontist, preferably one who is trained and experienced in early intervention.

Braces in Elementary School . . .

what's the Deal?

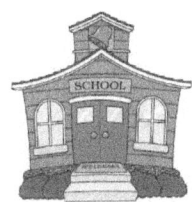As I mentioned, years ago orthodontics was only considered necessary for teenagers and some adults. By delaying orthodontic treatment until the teenage years, a majority of a patient's growth was completed, leaving very little that an orthodontist could do to correct jaw alignment and bite problems. As a result, there are many adults today who have had permanent teeth removed because there simply wasn't enough room in which

to fit all their teeth. Not only can having permanent teeth removed be a traumatic experience, the removal of permanent teeth may lead to premature facial aging as the upper front teeth, which support the lips, are moved backward in the face, resulting in less fullness of the lips. Temporary measures to support the lips, such as Botox and collagen, can't compare to the facial support offered by a full, natural-looking smile in which all the permanent teeth are present. Furthermore, there are adults today with extensive tooth wear, gum recession, and even headaches and jaw pain because their bite couldn't be corrected due to jaw misalignment. Fortunately, all of that has changed, as today's orthodontists have a much better understanding of jaw growth and development. Research has shown that there are actually two major growth spurts that your child will experience. The first accelerated growth period is known as the *preadolescent* growth spurt and usually occurs between eight and ten years of age. The final acceleration, known as the *adolescent* growth spurt, occurs around twelve to thirteen for most girls and around fourteen to sixteen for most boys. By taking advantage of the preadolescent growth spurt, many times we are able to create sufficient room for all of the adult teeth and align the jaws so that permanent tooth removal and jaw surgery may be avoided. It is important to understand that the timing of interceptive orthodontics is critical, as there is a small "*window of opportunity*" to take advantage of the preadolescent growth spurt. The primary difference between interceptive and adolescent orthodontics is that the majority of the baby teeth are still present during interceptive orthodontics. Treatment must be initiated before baby molar teeth are loose or the effectiveness of the treatment is greatly reduced. This is why an early evaluation is so important!

Perhaps one of the greatest *side effects* of early treatment is the enhanced self-esteem and confidence that every child experiences as their teeth are aligned and their smile improved. An unfortunate reality of today's high-tech world is the advent of cyber bullying, and we have found that for many young children an unattractive smile, such as big spaces or buckteeth, can make them a target for bullies both at school and online. While I have focused primarily on correcting a child's orthodontic problems over the years, tearful, appreciative parents have told me how much our early treatment has changed their son's or daughter's life. I hear stories of improved self-confidence, new friends, better grades, and happier kids! Many moms have told me that having their child go into middle school with a beautiful smile was more than worth what they paid to correct their child's orthodontic issues.

Is Early Treatment Really Necessary?

Although the American Association of Orthodontists recommends an evaluation for all children by age seven, early treatment is not without some controversy. There are some older or less progressive or less experienced orthodontists who think that interceptive orthodontics is unnecessary or only needed in very limited circumstances. These particular doctors will tend to extract permanent teeth more frequently (which could prematurely age your child's face) or push the teeth so far forward to uncrowd them that the patient can't close their lips comfortably. Perhaps even worse, these misinformed orthodontists start orthodontic treatment on children during a period that I call **no-man's-land** (growth-wise)—after the preadolescent growth spurt but before the adolescent growth spurt. To address the crowding issues, these orthodontists place and remove the braces before all the permanent teeth are erupted, which means that your child's bite will never be completely corrected, which could lead to further problems in the future that may, unfortunately, require more braces.

Another problem with starting orthodontics in no-man's-land is that there is usually considerable jaw growth remaining after the braces are removed, especially in boys, who tend to grow later and longer than girls. As the jaw grows, the teeth move with it, causing an imbalance in the previously aligned bite. This instability can lead to tooth shifting or crowding, tooth wear and gum recession, and, yet again, more braces! I am amazed at how many adults we retreat who have had at least one set of braces and still have crooked teeth and bite problems.

By taking care of growth issues early in children who need interceptive orthodontics, we are able to delay comprehensive orthodontics to finalize bite correction until jaw growth is no longer a factor for most patients. Early treatment allows us to determine the *right* time to start orthodontics so your child will not only have a beautiful smile but also a healthy, comfortable bite that will stand the *test* of time.

Signs that you or your child may need orthodontics

- Protruded upper front teeth (buckteeth)

- Overbite: upper front teeth too far forward of lower front teeth

- Underbite: lower front teeth biting ahead of upper front teeth

- Open bite: vertical space between upper and lower front teeth

- Crossbite: upper back teeth biting inside of lower back teeth

- Jaws that are too far forward (protrusion) or too far backward (retrusion)

- Thumb sucking or finger sucking

- Frequent headaches

- Jaw clicking or locking

- Impacted teeth

- Crowded or misaligned teeth

- Excessive tooth wear or gum recession

- Early loss of baby teeth or missing permanent teeth

- Difficulty chewing

What if My Child Isn't Ready for Braces?

Even though we have stressed the importance of an early eval-

uation for all children, the reality is that many of the condi-

tions present in your child's mouth may not need immediate

attention. If this is the case, it's still important to continue to

work with an orthodontist who will monitor your child's jaw

growth and development and assess the eruption of the adult

teeth to determine the optimal time to begin orthodontics to

correct the problems that have been discovered. Ongoing, pe-

riodic orthodontic checkups are a part of a healthy lifestyle.

Ideally, your child should continue to have regular assessments

with the orthodontist every six to twelve months. The best

practice when it comes to putting braces on a child's teeth is to

do it at the ideal time. The only way to pinpoint the ideal time is to continue with regular orthodontic evaluations. Most orthodontists will provide complimentary exams, so you don't need to worry about incurring an orthodontic bill every six to twelve months. Not only is it in the best interest of your child to put braces on at the *ideal* time, but it is also for the orthodontist as well. When we can zero in on the ideal time, it will end up saving us valuable chair time and reducing the overall length of the treatment, which helps to keep costs down as well. This is an important benefit because less treatment time helps to minimize damage to the teeth, such as cavities or decalcification (permanent white spots), gum disease, sore teeth, and all the other problems that can occur when braces are left on the teeth too long.

A Great Investment

The benefits of excellent orthodontic treatment are many. They include everything from an amazing smile and increased self-confidence to a decreased chance for periodontal disease and even heart disease. Straight teeth are easier to clean, so orthodontics lessens the chance of tooth decay or gum disease later in life. Having straight teeth and a healthy bite is one of the best ways to ensure that you keep your teeth for life. The good news is that orthodontics is faster, more aesthetic, and more comfortable than ever before! High quality orthodontic treatment is one of the best investments you can make and will pay huge dividends years after the braces are removed.

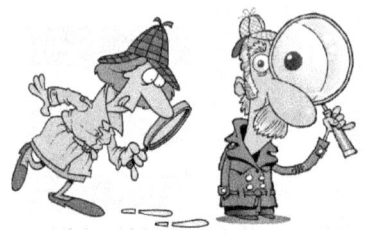

Finding an Orthodontist: The *Right* Choice Makes all the Difference

"**A**n orthodontist is one of the first healthcare professionals that will make treatment decisions that will affect how your child will look for the rest of their life," according to Dr. David Sarver, an orthodontist and a leading authority in smile design and facial aging. Finding the *right* orthodontist is no small feat and should not be taken lightly, as the consequences of your choice can last a lifetime. Some patients are fortunate enough to have a dentist or a friend refer them to a specific orthodontist. Others are told by their dentist that they need to see an orthodontist and then are given a handful of business cards from local ortho- dontists and left to make the decision on their own, a daunt- ing task to say the least! Regardless of how you are referred, there are several considerations when making your choice.

Education and Training of the Orthodontist

A major factor is the education of the orthodontist. Prior to their training, all orthodontists in the United States are re- quired to successfully complete four years of dental school

before enrolling in an orthodontic program. So all orthodontists are dentists, but not all dentists are orthodontists.
Admission to an accredited orthodontic program is highly
competitive and only about 5 percent of all dentists become orthodontists. The typical training program is two
to three years beyond dental school and covers a myriad
of topics in the graduate-level basic sciences, from head-
and-neck anatomy, radiography, child growth and development, bone physiology, embryology, craniofacial biology,
oral pathology, genetics, and even statistics. More specific
topics include the diagnosis and treatment of dentofacial
abnormalities, cephalometrics, orthodontic biomechanics,
dentofacial orthopedics, surgical orthodontics, and orthodontic techniques. A significant portion of the curriculum

is devoted to clinical orthodontics, allowing the orthodontic resident to develop proficiency through a broad, diverse experience in patient care. This clinical experience is invaluable and is what sets orthodontists apart from general dentists who *dabble* in orthodontics for some of their patients. Under the supervision of seasoned and experienced instructors, orthodontic residents learn what techniques work and what steps should be taken if orthodontic treatment does not proceed as planned.

But an orthodontist's education shouldn't stop there. With all of the developments and changes taking place, the practice of orthodontics is rapidly evolving. You want to find an orthodontist who is on top of the latest advancements. A good orthodontist is a consummate student, always reading about the latest developments and always improving his or her knowledge and service by attending continuing education courses and routinely training his or her team. But beware, not all new developments are what they claim, and there are instances where tried-and-true techniques are still the best way to go. An experienced orthodontist will be able to sort the wheat from the chaff.

Perhaps one of the most overlooked areas in orthodontics is the diagnosis and treatment of temporomandibular disorders or TMJ. Most residencies will cover the topic, but few will spend clinical time in the treatment of this many times debilitating disorder. There is an ongoing debate as to whether the bite or occlusion has anything to do with TMD. Most of the research is, in my opinion, self-serving and concludes that orthodontics does not *cause* TMJ. But that's not the right question. If orthodontists can

fix your bite, then why hasn't the incidence of TMJ among orth-

odontic patients decreased? I believe the answer is in how most

orthodontics is performed. Many years ago, I had the privilege of

attending the prestigious Roth-Williams Center for Functional

Occlusion in San Francisco. Functional occlusion* is a fifty-cent

word for orthodontics that establishes *harmony* between a stable

jaw joint position (the foundation of your jaws) and the bite. The

center was founded by Dr. Ronald Roth, who applied the same

techniques to orthodontics that a prosthodontist, or a restorative

dentist, uses to place crowns on all of the teeth in the mouth to

rebuild a damaged bite. After all, there is little difference between

moving every tooth in a patient's mouth with braces and chang-

ing the bite by placing crowns on every tooth! Each postgraduate "student" at the Roth-Williams center is an experienced ortho-

dontist and receives advanced training in the diagnosis and treat-

ment of TMJ and bite disorders over a two-year period. There

are hundreds of Roth-Williams graduates throughout the coun-

try and around the world who have helped tens of thousands of

patients eliminate their headaches and achieve beautiful, stable

smiles that stand the test of time.

> *Please note that there are orthodontists who use the term functional orthodontics but in no way practice the techniques prescribed by Drs. Roth and Williams. In fact, they do just the opposite, employing appliances that dislocate the jaw rather than place the jaw joint in a stable position. So beware!*

The Orthodontist's Experience

It's been said that experience is the best teacher, and when it

comes to orthodontics, nothing could be more valid. With a

good education, an orthodontist can be an excellent theoretician; with experience, an orthodontist becomes a great clinician. A Hindu proverb that I recently read comically makes the point, *"No physician is really good before he has killed one or two patients."* While I'm certain that nobody dies because of orthodontics, one of the biggest challenges to young orthodontists with all of their newly developed knowledge and skill is to know what works and what doesn't. After all, it usually takes about two to three years at a minimum for most inexperienced orthodontists to finish a case. After that, it takes at least another year or two to see what *holds up* in order to understand what works and what doesn't for a particular technique. And while that's occurring, a young orthodontist is also learning how to run a business and manage a team. From my own experience, I can tell you that after more than twenty-five years of practice and over ten thousand successfully treated cases, I don't practice orthodontics anything like I was originally trained. And while experience is indeed a great teacher, an orthodontist who doesn't take time to critically review his or her results and continues to do the same thing he or she was originally taught may not be much better. So, when considering experience, make sure the orthodontist you choose has a great reputation for providing years and years of high quality, cutting-edge orthodontic treatment.

Can My Dentist Do Orthodontics?

Legally, any licensed dentist can perform orthodontic treatment as well as any other dental specialty. Dental students receive nominal

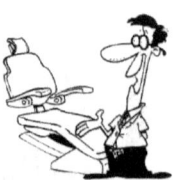

exposure to the specialty of orthodontics and almost no clinical experience. General dentists who elect to provide orthodontic services for their patients typically take a few weekend classes in a hotel and receive a very basic understanding of minor orthodontic tooth movement and, importantly, *no clinical experience.* Given the extremely brief training period, there is no time to review or learn any of the exhaustive lists of subjects and techniques that an orthodontist *must* learn. Because of the limited nature of their orthodontic education, most dentists rely on an outside consultant to plan the treatment for their patient. This is a rather disjointed approach to orthodontics, as the consultant rarely, if ever, has the opportunity to examine the patient in person. Some dentists will offer their patients all of their dental services *under one roof* and typically try to squeeze orthodontics between cleanings, fillings, dentures, root canals, and crowns. Just as your family physician would refer you to a cardiologist for a heart concern because of their expertise, an orthodontist limits the scope of his or her practice solely to providing quality orthodontic treatment for his or her patients. Given the far-reaching implications to a patient's appearance and health with orthodontic treatment, I would recommend that most patients seek their orthodontic care from an orthodontic specialist and limit the orthodontic treatment provided by general dentists to very minor movements of only a few teeth.

Your Orthodontic Experience!

Let's face it, orthodontic treatment can be disruptive to a busy schedule! In a typical orthodontic practice, to ensure quality and patient comfort, there are certain, more involved procedures that will require you to miss school or work. An efficient clinical team and a customer-oriented schedule will help minimize these interruptions to your day. A comfortable, well-designed office can also be essential to *on-time* scheduling as well. Unexpected or unplanned procedures, such as brace repairs, can also slow treatment and extend the time in braces, so it is critical that patients follow the orthodontist's instructions to the letter to avoid unnecessary delays. Perhaps the most important factor in the patient experience is the orthodontic team. The majority of orthodontic teams are women, and it's always nice to have a gentle touch whenever you're undergoing any kind of medical treatment, even something as easy as orthodontics. A highly trained, committed, and compassionate team is an essential part of your orthodontic care, as they work closely with your orthodontist and in fact will provide a large portion of the clinical treatment. A great team constantly trains and is always committed to its patient's success by using excellent clinical techniques and great communication skills. An excellent team is always focused on superb customer service and maintains a "can do" attitude at all times!

Beyond Straight Teeth

T here is so much more to orthodontics than straight teeth. An intriguing UC Berkeley thirty-year longitudinal study that examined the smiles of students in an old yearbook and then measured their well-being and success throughout their lives revealed some interesting findings. By measuring the smiles in the photographs, the researchers were able to predict how fulfilling and long lasting their marriages would be, how highly they would score on standardized tests of well-being and general happiness, and how inspiring they would be to others. The widest *smilers* consistently ranked highest in all the categories. British researchers found that one smile can provide the same level of brain stimulation as up to two thousand chocolate bars; they also found that smiling can be as stimulating as receiving up to sixteen thousand pounds sterling in cash. That's $25,000 a smile! Many people have been known to smile several hundred times per day. A typical fee for comprehensive orthodontic treatment ranges from $5,000 to $10,000. If you do the math, that's quite a *return on investment* throughout a person's lifetime!

In general, there are two major areas of focus for orthodontic treatment: aesthetics and function. Most of us aren't born with a *knockout* smile, and creating a beautiful smile requires careful consideration of several aesthetic factors combined with recognition of how the face changes with time. In their groundbreaking research, Drs. David Sarver and James Ackerman, leading authorities in smile design and facial aging, describe three areas of interest: macro-esthetics, mini-esthetics, and micro-esthetics. Macro-esthetics relates primarily to the appearance of the face and considers how the face grows and matures with time. Mini-esthetics correlates principally to all of the components around the mouth that create a beautiful smile. Finally, micro-esthetics focuses predominantly on the position, shape, and color of the teeth and gums. When these three aesthetic areas are *harmonized*, a beautiful smile is created!

Positive Aging and Orthodontics

When it comes to facial makeovers, most people think of plastic surgery. However, you may be surprised to learn that the shaping of a beautiful face can also be achieved by a well-trained orthodontist. Many people understand that orthodontists can straighten teeth but don't realize that these specialists can also influence facial growth to create an improved appearance that will last a lifetime unlike fillers and Botox, which must be *reapplied* periodically. Facial structures can be changed at any age; however, these alterations are especially effective for kids during growth spurts, particularly in those important teen years when self-image is beginning to form. New advancements in the field of orthodontics have enabled doctors to achieve remarkable aesthetic benefits as well as oral health improvements for patients in all stages of life. By predicting how the jaw and facial bones will grow, anticipating how the smile changes over time, and understanding the dynamic relationship between the teeth, lips, jaws, and other facial structures, an orthodontist can literally sculpt the face of the patient during treatment. It's not uncommon for parents to comment on the dramatic facial change we've been able to achieve for their child with interceptive ortho- dontics. Even adults report significant improvements in their face after completing orthodontic treatment. "Brace-lift" treatments can help adult patients look younger and feel more confident in their professional as well as their personal lives.

It's All about the Face! (Macro-esthetics)

A key concept when considering facial aesthetics is that of sym- metry. A balanced face with appropriate proportions is typically found more attractive by the opposite sex and by society in general. An astute orthodontist pays particular attention to the contours of the lower third of the face. They understand that the upper lip is supported by the teeth and how orthodontic movement of the teeth can affect the fullness of a patient's lips and even how much of their teeth they show when smiling. As a person ages, they tend to show less of their upper teeth and experience less fullness in the lips. *"If an orthodontist anticipates these changes, then treatment can be designed to provide a more youthful appearance for a longer time,"* says Dr. Sarver.

When the upper and lower jaws don't align properly, not only is the bite affected, but facial proportions are also unbalanced, which can detract from the appearance of one's face. For instance, a recessed lower jaw results in an overbite, where the upper front teeth are positioned ahead of the lower teeth, and a weak chin usually accompanied by sagging under the chin, or a double chin, which will become more evident with age. There are several ways to correct the overbite; however, the treatment plans can yield rather different results. One solution involves the removal of two upper teeth (one on either side) and pulling the upper front teeth backward into the extractions spaces. As the front teeth move backward, the overbite indeed will be corrected; unfortunately, as the front teeth move backward, the upper lip moves back and thins as well, since the upper front teeth no longer support the upper lip. Another more favorable way to correct the overbite would be to leave the upper front teeth in the forward position, which will maintain fullness in the upper lip, and then lengthen and advance the lower jaw surgically. As the lower jaw is moved forward, the overbite will also be corrected, and more importantly, as the chin advances, symmetry and balance is restored to the face, resulting in a stronger jawline and a decrease or elimination of the double chin. This is a perfect example of how one orthodontic plan can create facial *decline* and premature aging and another treatment can restore facial balance and actually turn back the hands of time!

Your Smile Matters! (**Mini-esthetics**)

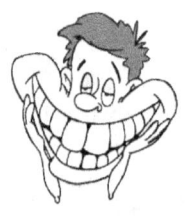 Next to jaw alignment, the two most important factors that determine the attractiveness of a smile are the width of the smile and the amount

of front teeth displayed, especially when smiling. Perhaps one of the greatest things we do for our patients at White Orthodontics is to give them a wide, natural-looking smile. We create these full smiles for a majority of our patients through a process known as palatal expansion. This procedure, which has been available since the 1960s, uses an orthodontic appliance known as an expander to widen the upper jaw. As the upper jaw is widened, the back teeth are moved outward as well, creating more room for crowded teeth and providing more support for the face. Not every orthodontist routinely uses palatal expansion. There are some orthodontists who never use palatal expansion and many who only use an expander when a crossbite, where the upper back teeth bite inside the lower, exists. Orthodontists who don't use expanders *attempt* to widen the smile by broadening the wires that connect the braces and pulling the teeth outward with rubber bands. Studies have shown that this approach only tips the teeth off of the bone, which is unstable, can create gum recession, and will impede bite correction as the back teeth flare out. Research also demonstrates that palatal expansion is much more effective in younger patients—yet another reason to have an early orthodontic evaluation for your children.

Show Your Stuff!

Have you ever noticed that when elderly people smile, you typically only see their lower front teeth and very little, if any, of their upper teeth? As a person ages, the lips thin and begin to droop and less and less of the upper front teeth are visible when smiling. For optimal aesthetics, a teenager should show the entire length of the upper front teeth and just a little bit of the gums above the teeth when smiling. This is critical for orthodontists and patients alike to understand. An aesthetically oriented orthodontist knows that the manner in which the braces are placed on the teeth and the *mechanics* that he or she employs can improve or even detract from the amount that the front teeth are displayed when smiling. I have consulted with many patients over the years who have had previous orthodontic treatment with other orthodontists and were unhappy with their results. In almost every case, the smile is too narrow, and in many of the cases, patients are actually showing less of their upper front teeth after orthodontics than before the braces. There is, however, a fine line to just how much of the gums should show above the teeth. Typically a few millimeters of gum is most aesthetic. After that, the smile can start to look *gummy* when an excessive amount of the gums is revealed. While it may look cute on an infant, a gummy smile on an adult may be viewed as unattractive. Fortunately, with proper planning, a gummy smile can be corrected with orthodontics, sometimes in conjunction with gum *sculpting* procedures.

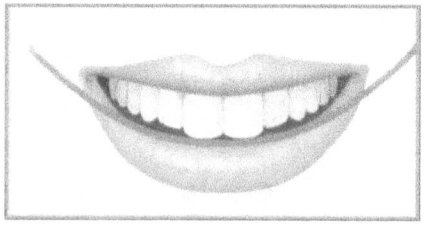

Figure 1: Smile Arc

Dr. Sarver also identified another major component of a beautiful smile—the smile arc. The smile arc is defined as the shape that is created by a line connecting the bottom edges of the upper front teeth. The most aesthetic smiles have a gentle curve connecting the bottom edges of the upper front teeth (from canine to canine) that is parallel to and almost touching the curvature of the bottom lip. With improper or inaccurate brace placement, a poorly trained orthodontist can actually flatten the smile arc or even create a reverse curvature of the smile arc, resulting in a less attractive smile.

Icing on the Cake! (Micro-esthetics)

Once facial balance and symmetry are established and a wide, natural-looking smile with a gentle smile arc is created, the shape and color of the teeth and gums must be considered before *finalizing* the smile. To some extent, a well-trained orthodontist with an eye for dental aesthetics can modify the shape of selected teeth to perfect the smile. However, many patients with a malocclusion can have extensive wear, or attrition of the teeth, due to an improper bite. In these instances, a restorative dentist can rebuild the previously worn teeth to the proper size and shape by using cosmetic bonding, veneers, or even porcelain crowns to put the *icing on the cake*, so to speak, and add the finishing touches to a beautiful smile. Worn teeth are more often seen in adults after years of jaw shifting and excessive pressure on the teeth from an improper bite. Fortunately, for most of our younger patients, having their bite properly corrected in their teens will save them a lifetime of pain and aggravation commonly seen with a malocclusion and also save them a lot of their hard-earned money by not having to have extensive restorative dentistry in their adult years. That is not to say that restorative dentistry is not needed for some teens who may have undersized or missing teeth. Interestingly, once their crooked and misaligned teeth have been straightened, they become more aware of discoloration or dullness in their teeth and choose to have cosmetic bleaching or whitening of their teeth to give their beautiful smile the sparkle and pizazz that really shows off their *investment*! Finally, gum sculpting procedures may be needed to uncover the full extent of some teeth that may be partially hidden under the gums. Sometimes patients are referred to a periodontist, or gum specialist, but many times we are able to painlessly sculpt the gums with a soft-tissue laser to enhance previously veiled smiles.

As you can see, there are many factors that contribute to a beautiful smile, and failure to identify these issues when planning orthodontic treatment can result in an unaesthetic result and an unhappy patient. I can't emphasize enough how important it is to find an orthodontist who understands these issues and routinely incorporates these concepts into his or her orthodontic treatment plan. Not all orthodontists achieve the same results, so *caveat emptor* (let the buyer beware)!

More Than You Can Chew?

You've heard the expression "don't bite off more than you can chew," but chewing is usually not the problem for most people. The difficulty for many patients results from what is known as *parafunction*, or clenching and grinding. People who clench or grind their teeth may experience premature tooth wear, shifting teeth, gum recession, and in extreme cases jaw clicking or popping, headaches, jaw locking, neck aches, tinnitus, or vertigo. Studies have demonstrated that these conditions may be caused by or aggravated by an improper bite. Almost every orthodontist discusses correcting the bite, but, surprisingly, very few do much to make it happen! As previously mentioned, functional orthodontists are specifically trained to diagnose and treat TMJ and bite disorders, establishing harmony between a stable jaw position and a correct bite. These doctors routinely screen for TMJ dysfunction during the initial orthodontic evaluation and *always* use instruments to quantify and track the jaw position. One of these instruments is called an articulator or bite simulator. An articulator allows the doctor to see the true bite with the jaw joints in their proper position. This instrument is routinely used by restorative dentists when given the task of rebuilding a patient's damaged bite. It may take a few extra steps for an orthodontist to use an articulator for all of his or her cases, but the information gained is invaluable and certainly worth the additional efforts! Many times an orthodontic case that seems straightforward when looking at a patient's bite in the mouth can suddenly become extremely complex when looking at the bite with the jaw in the proper position as it is with an articulator. Having this information before starting orthodontics allows the orthodontist to provide the appropriate treatment and ensure that the bite is fully corrected. Not having this valuable information before starting orthodontics can lead to serious complications that may result in extended treatment time or a dramatic change in the plan, such as requiring jaw surgery or, as in many cases, an incomplete result, which could ultimately require orthodontic retreatment in the future. Most orthodontists do not routinely use an articulator for their cases, but there are some who use them on the difficult ones. My question to them is how you know which ones are, in fact, difficult until you use the articulator!

Bio-Esthetic Smile Design

Through the years, I've seen people with an attractive smile still have problems because their bite was not properly corrected. It's very awkward to tell a patient with a nice smile that they need to wear braces again to correct their bite in order to remedy the problems they're experiencing. I've also observed patients with a stable, healthy bite but, unfortunately, a less-than-appealing smile. It's important to understand that a beautiful smile and a healthy bite are not mutually exclusive!

You can have it all, though. The answer is *Bio-esthetic smile design*. Bio-esthetic smile design is intended to provide *both* the beautiful smile that most people want and the healthy bite that every patient should have!

Beautiful Smiles for a Lifetime

A common frustration for orthodontist and patient alike is a phenomenon known as relapse. Orthodontic relapse is the tendency for previously crooked teeth to become misaligned again following orthodontic treatment. A long-term study conducted over sixty years by the University of Washington in Seattle reveals that the lower front teeth most frequently *recrowd* after the braces are removed. In our practice we intentionally place a custom-made permanent retainer behind the lower front teeth to help maintain their alignment. However, the best retainer is a perfect bite with a stable jaw position, which, as you have learned, takes more than just "lip service" to achieve. The jaw joint position is analogous to the foundation when building a house. One can have a beautiful house, but it will soon collapse without a stable foundation. The same is true for orthodontics, as a patient may complete treatment with an attractive smile only to see it fall apart or develop jaw pain if the jaw joints are not positioned properly. Functional orthodontists have a very clear set of goals that they strive to achieve for each of their patients, and a beautiful smile is only one part of a very complex puzzle. To preserve their stunning smile during and after orthodontics, patients are encouraged to maintain excellent oral hygiene and continue regular and periodic checkups and cleanings with their dentist while they're wearing braces. During treatment, patients are also urged to avoid hard or sticky foods that can damage the braces and sugary or acidic foods that can damage the teeth. Patients can also help retain their beautiful smiles by avoiding bad habits that will stress the teeth and jaw joints, such as nail biting, thumb sucking, and mouth breathing. The good news is that straight teeth are much easier to clean than crooked or misaligned teeth.

A Matter of Life and Breath

N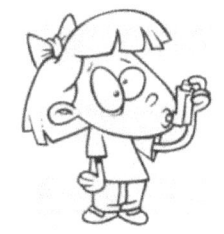ot to be overly dramatic, but your child may be slowing dying…and nobody knows it! Obstructive sleep apnea (OSA) affects an estimated fifteen million adult Americans and is present in a large percentage of patients with high blood pressure and other heart ailments, such as coronary artery disease, stroke, atrial fibrillation, and heart failure.

Sleep-disordered breathing (SDB) is a general term for breathing difficulties during sleep and affects approximately 4 to 11 percent of children. SDB can range from frequent loud snoring to obstructive sleep apnea (OSA), a condition involving repeated episodes of partial or complete blockage of the airway during sleep. When a child's breathing is interrupted while sleeping, the body experiences a reaction similar to choking. The heart rate slows, blood pressure rises, the brain is aroused, and sleep is disrupted. It's not uncommon for oxygen levels in the blood to drop, as well. Approximately 10 percent of children snore, and about 2 to 4 percent of the pediatric population has obstructive sleep apnea.

Could My Child Have OSA?

The most obvious symptom of sleep-disordered breathing is loud snoring at night. Breathing can be interrupted by a partial or complete blockage of the airway, resulting in gasping and snorting noises and a subsequent awakening from sleep. Poor sleep quality is frequently observed and may result in irritability, daytime sleepiness, hyperactivity, bedwetting, and difficulty concentrating in school. In addition to heart and lung ailments, children with sleep-disordered breathing may also experience slow growth and development due to a decrease in growth hormone production. SDB may also cause the body to have an increased resistance to insulin or daytime fatigue with decreases in physical activity, which can lead to obesity.

What Causes Sleep Apnea?

The most common cause of OSA is a small or narrow airway. The airway is basically formed by the throat, the soft palate, and the tongue. Changes in the size of the throat, and the position of the soft palate and tongue, can have a dramatic impact on the size of the airway. Obviously, the smaller the airway, the more difficult it is to breathe, especially during sleep, as the tongue tends to fall back into the airway as a person lies down and the muscles in the mouth and throat begin to relax.

Enlarged tonsils and adenoids will tend to decrease the airway shape and size and are a frequent cause of SDB. Another often overlooked cause of airway obstruction is the size and position of the tongue. Narrow upper and lower jaws, or a recessed lower jaw, tend to force the tongue downward and backward, thereby constricting and possibly obstructing the airway. A frequent cause of upper jaw narrowness is mouth breathing. Well-developed airways allow normal breathing through the nose with the mouth closed. Research has shown that air breathed through the nose is vastly superior for normal development than air breathed through the mouth.

A significant benefit to nasal breathing is the formation of nitric oxide in the sinuses, which is secreted into the nasal passages and inhaled through the nose. Nitric oxide is known to prevent bacterial growth and improves the lungs ability to absorb oxygen. During normal development, the bones of the face are shaped by a balance of muscular forces. Optimal breathing through the nose allows the tongue to be positioned up inside and to the front of the upper jaw. The tongue then exerts an expansive, outward, and forward pressure on the upper jaw and balances the constricting, or narrowing, pressure of the muscles of the cheeks and lips.

Primate studies have shown that obstructive nasal airways lead to open-mouth breathing. As the tongue assumes a lower position, the equilibrium of forces acting on the upper jaw is disrupted, and the muscles of the lips and cheeks exert an inward pressure on the teeth, creating a narrower, V-shaped upper jaw. The collapsed upper jaw, in turn, forces the tongue downward into the throat, thereby creating further airway obstruction. The narrower upper jaw creates not only overcrowding of the teeth but also a misalignment of the upper and lower jaws. Many times this results in an overbite and an open bite, where the upper front teeth protrude ahead of the lower front teeth and fail to overlap vertically.

The most frequent causes of mouth breathing are enlarged tonsils and adenoids, nasal obstruction, and environmental allergies. Whatever the cause, mouth breathing, unlike nasal breathing, allows unfiltered, cool air to irritate the tonsils and adenoids. In response, inflammation and swelling of the tonsils and adenoids occurs, resulting in further airway obstruction. It has been clearly demonstrated that obesity is a common cause of airway obstruction and sleep apnea in adults. However, research suggests that abnormal shape and position of the jaws is a much more important factor in determining who's at risk for developing sleep-disordered breathing in six- to eight-year-old children. Again, this is why an early evaluation by an "airway-aware" and properly trained orthodontist is so critical.

How Is OSA Diagnosed?

As with any disease or condition, a thorough diagnosis, including a comprehensive health history, is important. Symptoms such as loud snoring, mouth breathing, or school performance problems should be reported to your pediatrician, who can then make the appropriate referral. Ordinarily, an ENT specialist will become involved. My preference is to also have an evaluation by a *properly trained* dentist, pediatric dentist, or orthodontist, as many of the oral conditions that may contribute to OSA may go unrecognized by the medical professional.

The gold standard for testing for sleep-disordered breathing, either SDB or OSA, is the sleep study, or polysomnography (PSG). Wires are attached to the head and body to monitor brain waves, muscle tension, eye movement, breathing, and the level of oxygen in the blood. The test is usually administered in a sleep lab and is not painful but can occasionally produce inaccurate results, especially in children who may feel uncomfortable in a strange bed. Recently, an in-home sleep study has been developed in hopes of producing more accurate results in the confines of a more familiar place.

An orthodontic evaluation should also be performed to identify any skeletal imbalances or other conditions that could contribute to SDB. A lateral head x-ray has traditionally been used to assess the size of the airway and identify any possible narrowing or obstruction. With the advent of cone beam computed tomography (CBCT), a true three-dimensional analysis of the airway is now possible. Several sleep-disordered breathing questionnaires have proven to be quite accurate in determining who is suffering from SDB. When used in combination with a three-dimensional CBCT, the need for polysomnography has been eliminated in many cases.

Treatment for SDB

Enlarged tonsils and adenoids are the most common cause of SDB. A conservative approach using nasal rinses, decongestants, and steroid sprays is typically the first line of approach. If this regimen proves ineffective, surgical removal of the tonsils and adenoids (T&A) is generally considered. It may surprise you to learn that the majority of pediatric T&A procedures performed in the United States each year are done to treat sleep-disordered breathing and not for infections.

Another treatment protocol is the use of continuous positive airway pressure (CPAP), a mechanical device that applies mild air pressure in order to keep the airway open. CPAP is typically used by adults and sometimes in conjunction with T&A for severe OSA.

For those who cannot tolerate CPAP and are not a candidate for T&A, oral appliances can be made to force the lower jaw forward and temporarily open the airway. The appliance fits over the upper and lower teeth and is worn only at night while sleeping. The oral appliance is not without side effects; it can cause TMJ problems and shifting teeth, which may alter the bite. In adults where the jaws are no longer growing, surgical advancement and/or expansion of the upper and lower jaws may be necessary to open the airway.

Early Intervention Is a Must!

When it comes to orthodontics, *the biggest mistake a parent or family dentist can make is to wait until all the permanent teeth are in before having an orthodontic evaluation for your child*. By age seven, the majority of growth and development of the upper jaw is completed, and by age nine, the same holds true for the lower jaw. By age twelve, the majority of all facial growth is completed. Furthermore, if your child has an airway obstruction, the quality of their facial growth has been *negatively* impacted during most of their growth phase.

The longer one waits to intercede, the more severe the consequences and the more difficult the correction. Unfortunately, most orthodontists wait until the teenage years, when little facial growth remains, before attempting to correct what are, by now, longstanding problems. Sadly, the debate as to the effectiveness of early treatment continues in the orthodontic community while thousands of growing patients are harmed by what is referred to as "benign neglect," or "let's wait and see what happens."

What Can Be Done?

First and foremost, find an "airway-centric" orthodontist who recognizes the opportunity and the tremendous benefits that *properly designed* interceptive orthodontics can provide for growing patients. Previously in this book I described the benefits of upper and lower jaw expansion. In addition to creating a wider, more natural-looking smile and reducing the need for permanent tooth removal, palatal expansion creates more room for the tongue. As the palate widens, the tongue moves upward and forward to assume its proper position within the upper jaw. This forward movement of the tongue opens the airway. Since the floor of the nose is also the top of the upper jaw, the nasal cavity is also widened slightly, thereby decreasing nasal airway resistance and enhancing breathing.

A less common but likewise effective orthodontic treatment is the expansion of the lower dental arch. As the lower teeth are widened, the functional tongue space increases, further improving tongue posture and its positive influence on the airway.

There are some orthodontists who choose not to expand the jaws and instead have permanent teeth removed, which can further decrease the space for the tongue and actually constrict the airway. There are cases in which the dental crowding is so severe that permanent teeth need to be removed. In these cases, upper and lower arch expansion may be needed to mitigate the consequences of tooth removal.

Even the type of expander can have an impact on treatment. The bonded expander allows the jaw to rotate farther forward than a traditional expander, which may actually cause the lower jaw to rotate backward and possibly negate some of the benefits of expansion of the airway. More and more orthodontists are now considering the impact of the treatment they provide on their patients' airways. Some practitioners will also pre-scribe functional appliances, such as the Herbst or the MARA, which dislocate the lower jaw forward to correct an overbite. In theory, this should improve the overbite, but in reality these appliances, while popular, can create a false bite that can lead to TMJ problems.

In my opinion, *the most positive impact on a patient's airway is provided by jaw expansion and the subsequent improvement in tongue posture.* If a patient has an airway obstruction and sleep ap-nea due to a recessed chin, the optimal treatment is surgi-cal advancement of the lower jaw to correct the overbite and restore facial balance by creating a stronger profile. As the lower jaw is moved forward the tongue, which is attached to the lower jaw, is moved forward as well, thereby opening the constricted airway.

As stated at the beginning of this chapter, I don't want to be overly dramatic, but as you now know, undiagnosed and untreated airway obstruction can have a devastating and even possibly fatal impact on a person's health. As many older adults can tell you, when it comes to the body, unlike a fine wine, things don't usually improve with age. Many of our adult patients who require palatal expansion must have a surgical procedure to allow us to widen the jaws, which would have been unnecessary had *we* treated them when they were growing. Unfortunately, the majority of these patients did have braces as teenagers but did not have more comprehensive orthodontic treatment, including palatal expansion. Given the ease with which we can expand the jaws in growing patients, it only makes sense to have your child evaluated by age seven. This early assessment allows us to provide optimal orthodontic treatment at the most appropriate time.

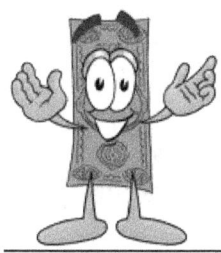

Paying for Orthodontics

One concern for many patients and parents is determining how to pay for orthodontics. While it can be a significant financial commitment for many families, it should be somewhat reassuring to know that even though the quality of care has improved dramatically, the cost of braces has actually declined on an inflation-adjusted basis since the 1960s. Given the *income bump* that people with a beautiful smile receive and all of the health benefits of a proper bite, high quality orthodontics is a smart investment any way you look at it. Perhaps the absolute worst way to shop for orthodontics is to find the cheapest or look for a deal. Just as with many services, you *do* get what you pay for! In order for an orthodontist to be profitable with a low fee, many of the things necessary for a great result have to be cut out and in turn the quality suffers. There is nothing more frustrating for a patient to endure than orthodontic *retreatment* because of a poor result, and there is nothing more painful than having to pay, yet again, for another set of braces.

Most importantly, an incomplete orthodontic diagnosis and inadequate treatment can lead to a lifetime of dental and medical problems costing tens of thousands of dollars and possibly shortening a person's lifespan. I see adult patients everyday who have gum recession, headaches, jaw clicking, and mouthfuls of crowns and bridges from worn down, broken, or lost teeth due to a bad bite even though they wore braces as a teen. It just makes sense to find the most thorough, best trained orthodontist who can give you not only a beautiful smile, but a healthy, stable bite as well. Spending a little bit more now, can save you tens of thousands of dollars and lots of pain and suffering years later!

Orthodontic Insurance

Insurance is one of the most common methods for paying for braces. It is important to understand that not all dental plans offer coverage for braces, but the right plan can help to defray a significant portion of the cost for braces. In choosing a dental insurance package, it is important to focus on finding a package that specifically covers orthodontists. The precise coverage provided will vary among plans, but many dental insurance plans will help to shave approximately 50 percent off the total cost of braces. In shopping for a dental plan, it should be understood that most plans will not provide coverage if the patient already has braces. Also, some plans require a waiting period, so it is important that you do not wait until treatment is necessary. Otherwise, you may find that treatment is not covered or that you need to delay treatment until the waiting period has passed.

Payment Plans

Even if you do not have dental insurance, some orthodontists will allow you to set up a payment plan. A payment plan works similar to installment plans for any other purchase and can help to make the cost of braces more affordable for many families.

Depending upon the orthodontist's requirements, you may need to make a down payment and then make monthly installments, many times interest free, over the duration of treatment. In most instances, treatment lasts about two years. Some orthodontists will even offer a discount if you are able to pay in full up front. This could help you to save several hundred dollars on the cost of braces.

Flex Spending Accounts (FSAs)

An FSA is a type of savings account set up by an employer for an employee; the account allows employees to contribute a portion of their regular earnings to pay for qualified expenses, such as medical expenses. One of the key benefits of a flexible spending account is that the funds contributed to the account are deducted from the employee's earnings before they are made subject to payroll taxes. As such, regular contributions to an FSA can significantly lower an employee's annual tax liabilities.

There are limits to how much can be contributed to an FSA account per year, and any funds left in the account at the end of the year are forfeited. One important factor to consider is that orthodontic treatment can last anywhere from one to three years and that the reimbursements for FSAs will only cover those expenses rendered during a plan year.

Third-Party Financing

Many families will use credit cards to pay for their orthodontic treatment. However, in times where interest rates on credit card balances may be rising, a dental services financing company that offers good terms may save patients money. Another attractive feature of third-party financing is the ability to extend payments beyond the length of the orthodontic treatment, thereby lowering the monthly payment amount even further. This is especially helpful for families with more than one family member in orthodontic treatment at the same time.

Orthodontic Charities

Low-income families can also sometimes qualify for help through orthodontic charities. The amount that one may be required to pay will depend upon his or her financial situation and the charity's guidelines. Accepted patients are often able to get orthodontic treatment at a low cost or even for free in some cases. Two well-known charities are Smiles Change Lives and Smiles for a Lifetime Foundation.

What's New in Orthodontics?

A frequent comment made by many of our parents who accompany their children to our office is "It's not fair! I wish my orthodontist had done it that way," followed by stories of four or five years of orthodontic *abuse*. I'm happy to report that orthodontic treatment has come a loooong way since the 1970s. Today's orthodontics is faster and more comfortable than ever. Perhaps the single greatest change has been in the braces themselves and in the wires that connect them:

Self-ligating braces: With the advent of dental bonding, the braces went from large metal bands that are shoved or tapped onto each tooth to a small metal bracket that is bonded directly to the teeth. With the first generation of brackets, the connecting wires are secured with small metal or elastic ties. This is still the most common brace in use today. The self-ligating bracket is the latest generation of braces in which the connecting wire is secured with a small heat-sensitive clip that is built into the bracket. This small clip eliminates the friction commonly found with the metal or elastic ties, allowing the teeth to align and move faster and more comfortably. For the aesthetically conscious, there are also self-ligating braces made out of porcelain for a less visible option and even braces that can be placed on the inside of the teeth for a completely invisible selection.

Heat-activated arch wires: The wire connecting the braces is known as the arch wire and is the moving or active part of the braces. Once the braces are placed on the teeth, they don't move; rather, it's the arch wire that provides the necessary pressure to move and align the teeth. Heat-activated metals were developed by NASA and are quite useful in orthodontics, as these arch wires are highly flexible at room temperature, allowing the wire to be placed and secured comfortably into misaligned braces. As the wire warms to body temperature, the force increases and the wire gradually returns to its original shape, thereby straightening the teeth. In the old days, the arch wires used were made out of rigid stainless steel, and the teeth were forced toward the wire over multiple and frequent tightening adjustments until the teeth were eventually aligned. Ouch!

Indirect bonding: Even though the braces don't move, it's critical that the brackets be placed accurately on the teeth. Most orthodontists place the braces directly on each tooth by hand *eyeballing* the approximate location of each bracket. While this technique can be effective for the front teeth, it can be quite inaccurate for the back teeth, as the lips, cheeks, and tongue can obscure the orthodontist's view. Indirect bonding allows the orthodontist to place the brackets on a model of the patient's teeth without the difficulties of placing the braces directly in the mouth. Once the brackets are set on the model, an elastic transfer tray (similar to an athletic mouth guard) is used to carry the braces from the model to the mouth. Not only are the braces placed more accurately, but also in less than half the time of direct bonding. Indirect bonding can also be completed virtually on computerized 3-D models.

Invisalign: Believe it or not, it is possible to move teeth without braces. Invisalign is a series of clear aligners, or plastic trays, that have the tooth movement built in to each subsequent aligner. The orthodontist or qualified dentist simulates the orthodontic treatment on a 3-D model until the teeth are straight, then a set of aligners are manufactured with these gradual movements incorporated into each successive clear tray. The benefits of Invisalign are that the trays are completely removable and that, since they are clear plastic, they are almost imperceptible. Typically the aligners are changed every two weeks as the teeth are gradually moved into place.

Expanders: Not so long ago, patients with crowded teeth had to have permanent teeth removed to create enough space to align the teeth. Unfortunately, this treatment option can lead to a flattening of the lips and profile for some patients. Today, space is typically created by enlarging the jaws with the use of expanders. Not only do expanders decrease the necessity for permanent tooth removal, but they also provide more support to the face and lips, thereby enhancing facial aesthetics and giving a more youthful appearance to patients as they age.

Digital impressions: If you hate having *goopy* impressions, or molds, made of your teeth, then you're in luck! Optical scanners and 3-D printers are on the verge of replacing those chalky mouthfuls. An optical scanner makes thousands of tiny pictures of your teeth to create a 3-D model. Recent advances in technology have created scanners that are faster and more accurate than ever before. A typical mouth can be comfortably scanned in five minutes or less.

Cone-beam computed tomography (CBCT): A CBCT scan provides an incredibly detailed and accurate three dimensional view of a patient's teeth and jaws. The CBCT is the dental version of a hospital CT scan with similar accuracy but significantly less radiation. This detailed 3-D scan allows the orthodontist to accurately plan treatment by getting a much clearer understanding of jaw misalignment, impacted teeth, jaw joint problems, and other conditions that may be missed on a regular 2-D X-ray.

Suresmile: The arch wires that connect the braces ultimately determine the final position of each tooth. Traditionally, an orthodontist adjusts or bends the wires by hand until the teeth are in their correct position. This technique involves a surprising amount of guesswork and will vary, of course, based on the skill of the orthodontist. Suresmile technology involves optical scanning, CBCT, and computerized robotics to create customized arch wires for each patient that virtually eliminates the *guesswork* of traditional orthodontics.

Insignia: Similar to suresmile, Insignia is a software program that allows an orthodontist to tailor the treatment for each patient. Using 3-D software and a proprietary process, *customized* braces and arch wires are created for each patient to provide precise treatment in less time.

Faster, Faster, Faster!

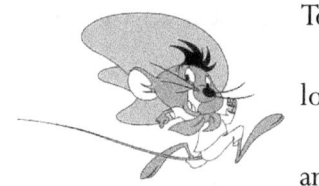 Today's orthodontic patients are looking for great smiles in the least amount of time, and the orthodontic profession has responded with several treatment *accelerators* in addition to the advances in brace and wire designs:

Wilckodontics: Tooth movement occurs when pressure applied to the teeth by braces is transferred to the surrounding bone. Procedures that enhance the response of the bone to the pressure will increase the speed of tooth movement. The first procedure to enhance bone response is Wilckodontics, which was introduced in 1998. Wilckodontics is a surgical procedure performed by periodontists and is completed soon after the braces are placed. Once the gums are numbed, they are reflected or moved away from the teeth to expose the bone surrounding the teeth. Small perforations are created in the bone around the teeth and a bone grafting material is inserted before the gums are returned to their original position. A twofold to fourfold increase in tooth movement velocity has been reported.

Propel: Recently a much less invasive procedure known as micro-osteoperforation, or Propel, has been introduced to increase the speed of tooth movement. After the administration of a topical anesthetic, small perforations are placed between the teeth where accelerated movement is desired. A 40 percent increase in tooth movement has been demonstrated.

AcceleDent: A nonsurgical orthodontic enhancement that delivers gentle vibrations, or micropulses, to the teeth. A mouthpiece is worn for twenty minutes each day to increase bone remodeling, thereby accelerating tooth movement. Treatment velocity is increased by 50 and it has also been reported that orthodontic treatment is more comfortable as well.

A Word of Caution . . .

Perhaps the most popular innovation in recent years in orthodontics to correct overbites has been the functional appliance. Claims have been made that functional appliances cause the lower jaw to grow more, but the research has only demonstrated an acceleration, not an increase, in lower jaw growth. The concept with any functional appliance is that the lower jaw is forced forward with the jaw joints out of the socket in order to "stimulate" jaw growth.

Herbst appliance/MARA appliance/Twin Block appliance: Two of these appliances are glued in place and one is removable. All of them are designed to force the lower jaw forward, moving the jaw out of its socket. As a functional orthodontist, I have spent my entire career helping people eliminate their pain or creating a stable bite for the majority of my patients by concentrating on seating the jaw in its correct position in the socket. An appliance that purposely *dislocates* the jaw is a major concern for me, and although a very popular appliance in our profession, I would urge caution when considering it.

Let the Journey Begin!

Hopefully, by now, you understand the many benefits of orthodontic treatment from an amazing smile and increased self-confidence to a decreased chance for periodontal disease and even heart disease. As I mentioned, straight teeth are easier to clean, so orthodontics lessens the chance of tooth decay or gum disease later in life. Having straight teeth and a healthy bite is one of the best ways to ensure that you keep your teeth for life.

Fortunately, today's orthodontic treatment is faster, more aesthetic, and more comfortable than ever before!

Where will your orthodontic journey take you? Attractive television anchor, saleswoman of the year, Fortune 500 CEO, high-powered attorney-with the health and confidence that a new smile will give you, the possibilities are endless! As you begin your journey, I hope you will find this book to be helpful. You now know what questions to ask and what qualities to look for when searching for an orthodontist. Don't forget, "if you don't know where you're going, any road will get you there"! So choose wisely. As I said at the outset, I truly believe that quality orthodontic treatment is one of the best investments anyone can make, and I hope you'll choose to make an investment with *guaranteed* returns for you or someone in your family. Best of Luck!

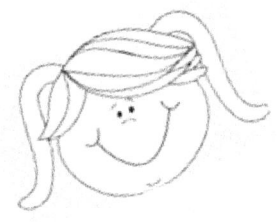

Fun Facts about Smiles . . .

- **Forcing yourself to smile can boost your mood:** Psychologists have found that even if you're in bad mood, you can instantly lift your spirits by forcing yourself to smile.

- **It boosts your immune system:** Smiling really can improve your physical health, too. Your body is more relaxed when you smile, which contributes to good health and a stronger immune system.

- **Smiles are contagious:** It's not just a saying! Smiling really is contagious, scientists say. In a study conducted in Sweden, people had difficulty frowning when they looked at other subjects who were smiling, and their muscles twitched into smiles all on their own.

- **Smiles relieve stress:** Your body immediately releases endorphins when you smile, even when you force it. This sudden change in mood will help you feel better and release stress.

- **It's easier to smile than to frown:** Scientists have discovered that your body has to work harder and use more muscles to frown than it does to smile.

- **It's a universal sign of happiness:** While handshakes, hugs, and bows all have varying meanings across cultures, smiling is known around the world and in all cultures as a sign of happiness and acceptance.

- **Smiling helps get you promoted:** Smiles make a person seem more attractive, sociable, and confident, and people who smile more are more likely to get a promotion.

- **Smiles are the most easily recognizable facial expression:** People can recognize smiles from up to three hundred feet away, making it the most easily recognizable facial expression.

- **Women smile more than men:** Generally, women smile more than men, but when they participate in similar work or social roles, they smile the same amount. This finding leads scientists to believe that gender roles are quite flexible. Boy babies, though, do smile less than girl babies, who also make more eye contact.

- **Smiles are more attractive than makeup:** A research study conducted by Orbit Complete discovered that 69 percent of people find women more attractive when they smile than when they are wearing makeup.

- **Babies start smiling as newborns:** Most doctors believe that real smiles occur when babies are awake at the age of four to six weeks, but babies start smiling in their sleep as soon as they're born.

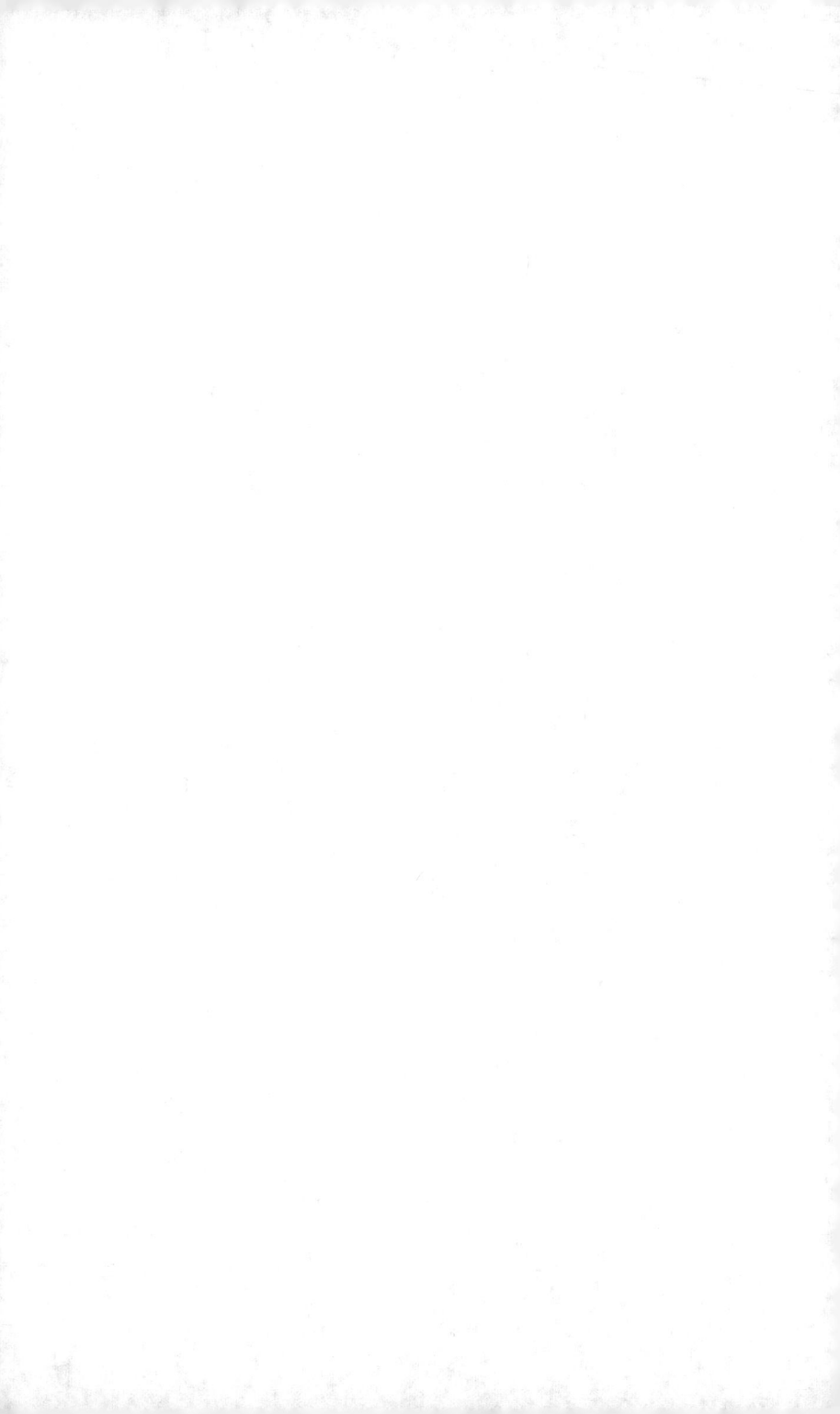